THE EASY 5-INGREDIENT

MEDITERRANEAN DIET COOKBOOK

FOR TWO

Quick and Healthy Recipes Designed for Couples on a Journey to Harmony and Shared Moments

Adam C.

DEDICATION

This book is dedicated to all my Readers

CONTENTS

Chapter 1: Introduction

Cooking is more than just a ritual; it's an adventure that you do together, a delicious taste test, and a symbol of your bond with another person. When it comes to culinary explorations, the Mediterranean Diet is particularly noteworthy for its capacity to strengthen bonds between partners as well as for its health benefits. Together, the flavors create a symphony of flavors that evoke special memories. This is "The Easy 5-Ingredient Mediterranean Diet Cookbook for Two: Quick and Healthy Recipes Designed for Couples on a Journey to Harmony and Shared Moments."

1.1 Why the Mediterranean Diet?

The people who live in the Mediterranean region embrace the Mediterranean Diet as a way of life rather than merely a set of recipes. This dietary pattern, which is well-known for enhancing heart health, longevity, and general well-being, places an emphasis on fresh, whole foods that are abundant in fruits, vegetables, whole grains, lean proteins, and healthy fats especially olive oil. Bright, sun-kissed vegetables and basic ingredients that let the natural tastes show through are the cornerstones of this dish.

However, why would a couple adopt the Mediterranean diet? It provides a communal experience that goes beyond the dinner table in addition to the health advantages. It's about enjoying every taste, the bonding experience of cooking a meal together, and the satisfaction of feeding your body healthful foods. When you adopt this lifestyle as a couple, cooking and sharing scrumptious, nourishing meals together not only strengthens your bond but also invests in your health.

1.2 Benefits of Cooking Together

Cooking together is a dynamic and fulfilling experience that extends beyond the plate of food. Here are a few strong advantages:

1. Bonding and Communication: The kitchen is turned into a place where people may freely communicate and work together. Together, while you chop, sauté, and stir, you get experience overcoming obstacles, delegating tasks, and acknowledging accomplishments. It's a strengthening event that strengthens the basis of your partnership.

2. Quality Time: It might be difficult to find quality time in the fast-paced world of today. Together, and away from outside distractions, cooking offers a concentrated moment for connection. It's a chance to have deep conversations and make treasured memories.

3. Learning and Developing Together: In the kitchen, there's always something new to learn, regardless of experience level. A sense of mutual learning and development is fostered by attempting new dishes, experimenting with flavors, and conquering culinary challenges with one another.

4. Healthier Selections: Since you are in charge of the ingredients when you cook at home, you can choose healthier options. With its focus on nutrient-rich meals, the Mediterranean Diet promotes both spouses' general health and wellbeing.

5. Culinary Creativity: Your ingredients are your palette, and the kitchen is your canvas. Cooking with others fosters creativity since it allows you to customize recipes to your own tastes and try different flavors, textures, and presentation styles.

1.3 Setting the Stage for Culinary Harmony

There's more to creating a peaceful cooking atmosphere than simply assigning someone to chop the vegetables or man the burner. It's about encouraging an environment of mutual respect, communication, and shared accountability. Here's how to create the ideal environment for harmonious cooking:

1. Interaction is Crucial: Openly talk about your food planning, tastes, and any dietary requirements. By avoiding misunderstandings and ensuring that everyone is on the same page, effective communication enhances the enjoyment of cooking.

2. Give thoughtful assignments: Assign work in accordance with each person's interests and areas of strength. Assigning tasks appropriately makes the process efficient and pleasurable, for example, if one person enjoys slicing veggies while the other is great at grilling.

3. Celebrate Your Success: Congratulate each other on your culinary accomplishments, whether it's grilling a piece of salmon to perfection or creating the right taste balance in a salad. Recognizing the work that went into the food improves the experience as a whole.

4. Establish a Calm Ambience: While cooking, turn on your preferred music, light some candles, or pour a glass of wine. Creating a calm environment makes the kitchen a sanctuary where you can decompress, spend time with each other, and relish the pleasure of cooking together.

Every recipe in this cookbook is created with simplicity in mind; they are all simple to make, call for just five ingredients, and are meant to serve two people. May the times spent together in the kitchen provide you happiness, nourishment, and a stronger bond as you set off on this culinary adventure. Prepare to be pleasantly surprised by the simplicity and joy of the Mediterranean Diet as a pair, building a path to harmony and quality time together one mouthwatering meal at a time.

Chapter 2: Understanding the Mediterranean Diet

Starting a Mediterranean diet is more than just following a few recipes; it's a way of life that encompasses a wide range of tastes, health advantages, and cultural customs. The fundamentals of the Mediterranean diet are covered in this chapter, setting the stage for couples to enjoy a delicious culinary journey with "The Easy 5-Ingredient Mediterranean Diet Cookbook for Two: Quick and Healthy Recipes Designed for Couples on a Journey to Harmony and Shared Moments."

2.1 Fundamentals and Ideas

The historic dietary practices of the nation's bordering the Mediterranean Sea serve as inspiration for the Mediterranean Diet, which is a flexible and sustainable eating plan rather than a strict set of restrictions. Fundamentally, this diet is defined by the following guidelines:

1. Plenty of Plant-Based Foods: Fruits, vegetables, whole grains, legumes, nuts, and seeds should make up the majority of your meals. These nutrient-dense meals are high in antioxidants, fiber, vitamins, and minerals.

2. Healthy Fats: Olive oil is a great source of healthy fats. A mainstay of the Mediterranean diet, olive oil contains monounsaturated fats that are associated with heart health.

3. Moderate Dairy and Poultry Consumption: Consume lean poultry and dairy in moderation, ideally in the form of yogurt and cheese. Consume less red meat and give fish and seafood first priority.

4. Spices and Herbs: Instead of using salt to flavor your food, use spices and herbs. This improves the flavor while also offering more health advantages.

5. Social Eating: Eating is supposed to be a communal activity. Around the table, spend time with those you love, enjoy the meal, and the company of one another.

6. Moderate Red Wine Consumption: Although not required, a hallmark of the Mediterranean lifestyle is the moderate use of red wine, especially at meals. Alcohol shouldn't be a part of your lifestyle if it isn't already.

Comprehending these tenets furnishes a guide for formulating delectable dishes that conform to the health-conscious customs of the Mediterranean area.

2.2 Key Ingredients and Pantry Essentials

Investing in fundamental foods and pantry staples that serve as the foundation for this culinary adventure is crucial if you want to make the Mediterranean Diet a reality in your kitchen. Here are a few essentials:

1. Olive oil: An essential component of the Mediterranean diet, olive oil gives food richness and complexity. Because extra virgin olive oil has more nutrients and a stronger flavor, go for it.

2. Fresh Produce: Stuff a rainbow of fresh fruits and veggies into your trolley. Vegetables with a wide range of uses include citrus fruits, peppers, tomatoes, cucumbers, and leafy greens.

3. Whole Grains: Opt for whole grains including brown rice, quinoa, bulgur, and farro. These grains offer a variety of vital minerals as well as fiber.

4. Legumes: Chickpeas, lentils, and beans are great providers of fiber and plant-based protein. They go well with soups, stews, and salads.

5. Nuts and Seeds: Nuts like flaxseed, chia seeds, walnuts, and almonds give foods a crunch and nutritious boost. Add them to yogurt or sprinkle them over salads.

6. Lean Protein: Consume skinless chicken and fish, particularly fatty varieties like mackerel and salmon. These protein sources provide good fats and necessary elements.

7. Dairy: For their rich flavors and adaptability, go for feta cheese and Greek yogurt. They work well in savory as well as sweet recipes.

8. Herbs and Spices: Assemble a collection of spices and herbs, such as cumin, thyme, basil, oregano, and rosemary. These improve food flavors without using a lot of salt.

9. Whole-Wheat Bread and Pasta: Select whole-wheat bread and pasta variations. When compared to processed grains, they provide more minerals and fiber.

Having these ingredients on hand makes it easy to prepare flavorful and nourishing Mediterranean dinners for two.

2.3 Health Benefits for Couples

In addition to its delicious flavors and rich culinary traditions, the Mediterranean Diet has several health advantages that make it a great option for couples who want to put their health first. The following are some of the main health benefits:

1. Heart Health: Eating a diet high in nuts, seafood, and olive oil promotes heart health. Omega-3 fatty acids from fish and the monounsaturated fats in olive oil have been related to a decreased risk of heart disease.

2. Weight control: Eating a lot of fruits, vegetables, and whole grains increases satiety; this makes it simpler to keep a healthy weight. The diet's emphasis on foods high in nutrients also benefits general nutrition.

3. Decreased Inflammation: Many Mediterranean foods, including fatty fish and olive oil, have anti-inflammatory qualities that may help lower inflammation in the body. Arthritis and heart disease are two conditions that are linked to chronic inflammation.

4. Better Blood Sugar Control: Eating foods high in fiber and consuming whole grains in moderation will help improve blood sugar regulation and lower the risk of type 2 diabetes.

5. Brain Health: Including fish, which is high in omega-3 fatty acids, has been linked to positive effects on cognition. Reduced risk of neurodegenerative disorders and cognitive decline has been associated with the Mediterranean diet.

6. Cancer Prevention: Antioxidants from fruits and vegetables, one of the Mediterranean diet's constituents, have been linked to a decreased risk of developing some types of cancer. The beneficial advantages of the diet may be attributed to its overall focus on whole, minimally processed foods.

7. Longevity: Research has indicated a higher chance of longevity when following the Mediterranean diet. Overall longevity is influenced by the combination of a healthy lifestyle and a well-balanced food.

Adopting the Mediterranean Diet as a pair not only paves the way for great meals but also for a joint dedication to wellbeing and health. Not only are you feeding your bodies with these concepts, but you're also cultivating a lifestyle that promotes longevity and vitality.

We'll look at how to make these ideas and ingredients into delicious dinners for two in the next chapters. Prepare to delight in the simplicity and richness of the Mediterranean Diet from breakfast to dinner and every snack in between, all while fostering a path to harmony and quality time spent with loved ones in the center of your kitchen.

Chapter 3: Kitchen Essentials for Two

The kitchen is the center of any house, and while cooking together, having the appropriate utensils, a well-organized workspace, and effective purchasing techniques may make the whole process more pleasurable and easy. We'll look at the kitchen necessities in this chapter, which will help you prepare easy, nutritious meals for two, following the guidelines in "The Easy 5-Ingredient Mediterranean Diet Cookbook for Two: Quick and Healthy Recipes Designed for Couples on a Journey to Harmony and Shared Moments."

3.1 Tools and Utensils

Getting your kitchen set up with the proper appliances and utensils is the first step to a peaceful kitchen. The following is a list of necessities to help your cooking adventure go more smoothly:

1. Premium Knives: Make a purchase of a set of premium knives, which should include a serrated knife, paring knife, and chef's knife. Sharp knives simplify the process of cutting and slicing food and improve cooking in general.

2. Cutting Boards: To avoid cross-contamination, keep a variety of cutting boards on hand, ideally color-coded for the various food groups. Select materials that require less upkeep and are easy to clean.

3. Mixing Bowls: To prepare and combine components, a variety of mixing bowls in different sizes is necessary. Choose dishes that are sturdy, safe to use in the microwave, and simple to clean.

4. Measuring Cups and Spoons: When cooking, precise measurements are essential. Invest in measuring spoons for accuracy as well as dry and liquid measurement cups.

5. Cookware: A multipurpose cookware set that includes a stockpot, saucepan, and non-stick skillet can be used for a variety of cooking tasks. When selecting cookware, take the size of your recipes into account.

6. Baking Sheets and Pans: Having high-quality baking sheets and pans is crucial, whether you're roasting veggies or making a delectable dessert. For simple clean up, opt for non-stick alternatives.

7. Utensils: Make sure you have a range of utensils, including wooden spoons, ladles, tongs, and spatulas. Using these instruments simplifies the process of handling various ingredient types and cooking techniques.

8. Blender or Food Processor: For making smoothies, sauces, and dressings, a blender or food processor comes in handy. Additionally, it can save time when cutting and pureeing ingredients.

9. Grater and Zester: Flavor your food with freshly grated cheese, zest from citrus, and spices. Having a good grater and zester is crucial if you want to use these in your food.

10. Can Opener: Although it can appear like a little tool, having a trustworthy can opener is essential for getting at foods like beans, tomatoes, and other pantry staples.

11. Colander: You may rinse canned products, wash vegetables, and drain pasta with a colander. Pick one that is easy to use and has strong grips.

12. Timer: Especially when multitasking, a kitchen timer is a basic yet very useful item. It guarantees that your food will be cooked to perfection without burning.

13. Storage Containers: You can keep leftovers and meal-prepped components effectively if you have a range of storage containers in various sizes. Choose microwave- and dishwasher-safe containers.

These basic tools will put you in a good position to tackle the dishes in this cookbook with confidence and ease.

3.2 Organizing Your Kitchen for Efficiency

Cooking harmony is mostly dependent on having a well-organized kitchen. The following advice will help you maximize the usable area in your kitchen:

1. Clear Countertops: To begin, clear your countertops of any debris. Just the necessities, such frequently used tools and equipment, should be kept. This makes the area hygienic and welcoming while also giving enough of space for meal preparation.

2. Group Related Items: Sort your kitchen utensils and gadgets according to their intended use. Pots, pans, and cooking tools should be kept close to the stove, while cutting boards, knives, and mixing bowls should be kept near the prep area.

3. Label and Sort Pantry things: Invest some effort in organizing your pantry by putting related things in one section. To distinguish basics like grains, legumes, and spices, use clear containers or labels. This facilitates finding ingredients when preparing meals.

4. Assign Storage Spaces: Set aside particular spaces for the storage of baking sheets, pots and pans, and small appliances. This simplifies the cooking procedure and facilitates keeping the kitchen organized.

5. Establish a Cooking Zone: Set aside a certain space for preparing food. Make sure your mixing bowls, knives, and cutting boards are easily accessible. Setting up a specific area for preparation work increases productivity and lessens the possibility of clutter.

6. Organizing Your Freezer and Refrigerator: Make sure you frequently check what's inside your freezer and refrigerator. Get rid of anything that have gone bad and arrange the shelves so they are accessible. To keep comparable goods together, think about use storage bins.

7. Meal Prep Station: Establish a dedicated meal prep station if there is room. This can comprise containers for prepared materials, a cutting board, and a set of knives. Quick meal assembly is made easier by a well-organized meal prep area.

8. Frequent Maintenance: Allocate a specific amount of time for routine kitchen upkeep. As needed, clear, clean surfaces, and wipe down appliances. This guarantees that your kitchen will always be a welcoming and useful area.

In addition to increasing productivity, a well-organized kitchen makes cooking as a pair more pleasurable.

3.3 Shopping Tips for Two

Effective and considerate grocery shopping is the cornerstone of a good dinner preparation. The following advice can help your food shopping trip go more smoothly and more efficiently if you're cooking for two:

1. Plan Your Meals: Make a weekly meal plan before you go to the grocery shop. This makes it easier for you to make a targeted shopping list and lowers the possibility that you would buy unnecessary things.

2. Purchase Seasonal and Fresh Produce: Whenever feasible, opt for seasonal and fresh produce. This not only guarantees that your ingredients are of the highest quality and flavor, but it also supports local farmers.

3. Shop the Periphery: The fresh produce, meat, dairy, and baked goods sections of most grocery shops are situated around the periphery. Prioritize whole, unprocessed foods by concentrating your purchasing on these areas.

4. Stock Up on Staples: Make sure your pantry is well-stocked with items that are essential to the Mediterranean diet, like whole grains, legumes, olive oil, canned tomatoes, and an assortment of herbs and spices. Preparing meals is more convenient when these supplies are available.

5. Purchasing in quantity: If there are certain pantry goods that you use regularly, think about purchasing in quantity. Long-term financial savings and fewer retail visits are possible with this.

6. Verify the Expiration Dates: To guarantee freshness, verify the expiration dates while buying perishable goods. This is crucial for products like dairy, eggs, and packaged foods in particular.

7. Be Mindful of Portions: Cooking for two means being mindful of portion sizes. Consider the shelf life of perishable items and buy quantities that you can reasonably consume before expiration.

8. Investigate Local Markets: For fresh, in-season produces, check out the local farmers' markets. This is not only a fun experience, but it also gives you a chance to meet local farmers and find unusual ingredients.

9. Consider Frozen Fruits and Vegetables: If you have ingredients that might go bad before you use them, you might want to think about freezing fruits and vegetables. They are practical for quick and simple meal preparation and maintain their nutritional worth.

10. Divide and Conquer: Split the shopping list between you and your shopping companion. This expedites the procedure and enables each person to concentrate on particular retail sections.

11. Keep Your Options Open: If a specific ingredient isn't available, don't be afraid to try something else. The Mediterranean diet is adaptable, and a lot of recipes may be changed according on what ingredients are available.

You can make grocery shopping easier and make sure your kitchen is well stocked with everything you need to prepare delicious Mediterranean-inspired dinners for two by adopting these shopping strategies into your daily routine.

Building your kitchen equipment collection, refining your buying tactics, and organizing your area are all contributing to the creation of a culinary adventure that will bring you joy, harmony, and shared moments while cooking scrumptious and nutritious meals together. We'll get into the core of this adventure in the future chapters recipes that are specifically created to celebrate the joy of cooking together and bring the tastes of the Mediterranean Diet to your table. Prepare to go on a delicious journey of shared experiences and flavors.

Chapter 4: Breakfast Delights

Breakfast is a holy ritual that couples share to connect, plan the day, and enjoy the first tastes of the day. It is the dawn of the day. This chapter features breakfast treats made for two that embody the principles of the Mediterranean diet. Not only are these recipes quick and simple, but they are also meant to give your morning a boost of vigor and energy, paving the way for a peaceful day filled with moments spent together.

4.1 Energizing Smoothie Bowls

Smoothie bowls are an energy-boosting and refreshing way to start the day. These bowls, which are loaded with antioxidants, vitamins, and minerals, not only wake you up but also give you a healthy start to the day. Smoothie bowls are so versatile that you may add your own fruits, nuts, and seeds to make them uniquely yours.

Ingredients:

- 1 cup frozen mixed berries (strawberries, blueberries, raspberries)

- 1 ripe banana
- 1/2 cup Greek yogurt
- 1 tablespoon honey
- Toppings: sliced almonds, chia seeds, fresh berries

Instructions:

1. In a blender, combine the frozen berries, banana, Greek yogurt, and honey.
2. Blend until smooth and creamy, adjusting the consistency with a splash of water or milk if needed.
3. Pour the smoothie into bowls and top with sliced almonds, chia seeds, and fresh berries.
4. Serve immediately and enjoy the vibrant burst of flavors.

This delightful smoothie bowl not only fuels your body with essential nutrients but also encourages creativity as you experiment with different fruit combinations and toppings. It's a breakfast treat that combines health and harmony in every spoonful.

4.2 Mediterranean Omelette for Two

An omelette with a Mediterranean flair will make your breakfast experience unforgettable. Fresh vegetable, herb, and feta cheese tastes abound in this omelette, which is a savory feast that transports the Mediterranean's sunny energy to your plate.

Ingredients:

- 4 large eggs
- 1 tablespoon olive oil
- 1/2 cup cherry tomatoes, halved
- 1/4 cup red bell pepper, diced
- 1/4 cup red onion, finely chopped
- 1/4 cup spinach, chopped
- 2 tablespoons feta cheese, crumbled
- Salt and pepper to taste
- Fresh basil for garnish

Instructions:

1. In a bowl, beat the eggs until well combined. Season with salt and pepper.
2. Heat olive oil in a non-stick skillet over medium heat.
3. Add cherry tomatoes, red bell pepper, and red onion to the skillet. Sauté until the vegetables are tender.
4. Pour the beaten eggs over the sautéed vegetables, ensuring they are evenly distributed.

5. Allow the eggs to set at the edges, then gently lift the edges with a spatula to let the uncooked eggs flow underneath.

6. Sprinkle chopped spinach and crumbled feta cheese over one half of the omelette.

7. Once the eggs are fully set, carefully fold the omelette in half.

8. Slide the omelette onto a plate, garnish with fresh basil, and serve hot.

A tasty and high-protein way to start the day is with this Mediterranean omelette. Together, the vibrant vegetable medley and the creamy feta cheese form a flavorful fusion that will leave you feeling energised and prepared to take on the day.

4.3 Quick and Healthy Granola Parfait

Enjoy a simple and nutritious granola parfait for a satisfying breakfast that tastes like a delight. A delicious symphony of textures and flavors is produced by the layers of Greek yogurt, fresh fruit, and handmade granola, which strikes the ideal balance between crunch and sweetness.

Ingredients:

- 1 cup Greek yogurt
- 1 cup mixed berries (strawberries, blueberries, raspberries)
- 1/2 cup granola (homemade or store-bought)
- 1 tablespoon honey
- Mint leaves for garnish

Instructions:

1. In serving glasses or bowls, start with a layer of Greek yogurt.
2. Add a layer of mixed berries on top of the yogurt.
3. Sprinkle a generous layer of granola over the berries.
4. Drizzle honey over the granola layer for a touch of sweetness.
5. Repeat the layers until you reach the top of the glass.
6. Garnish with a few fresh berries and mint leaves.
7. Serve immediately and enjoy the delightful crunch and creaminess of this parfait.

This granola parfait has a great blend of flavors and textures in addition to being aesthetically pleasing. This breakfast delight feels decadent, but it also neatly fits the Mediterranean Diet's nutritious guidelines.

As you enjoy these morning treats together, keep in mind that the act of breaking bread (or eggs) together in the morning is the first step toward harmony and shared moments. These recipes are designed to enhance your morning routine with flavors that speak to each other, whether it's the colorful vibrancy of a smoothie bowl, the savory embrace of a Mediterranean omelette, or the sweet crunch of a granola parfait. Prepare to bring the essence of the Mediterranean to your breakfasts and set out on a day full of conviviality and delicious food.

Chapter 5: Favorite Lunchtime Recipes

In the middle of the day, lunch is a chance to take a break, recharges, and spend time with your significant other. This chapter features lunchtime favorites that are perfect for two people and are all based on the colorful and healthful Mediterranean Diet. These dishes are designed to fuel your body and strengthen your bond as you travel toward harmony and shared moments, in addition to being quick and simple to prepare.

5.1 Greek Salad with Grilled Chicken

A traditional Mediterranean cuisine that epitomizes simplicity and freshness is Greek salad. This dish turns a simple side salad into a filling, high-protein meal for two by adding grilled chicken.

Ingredients:

- 2 boneless, skinless chicken breasts
- 1 tablespoon olive oil
- 1 teaspoon dried oregano
- Salt and pepper to taste
- 4 cups mixed salad greens
- 1 cup cherry tomatoes, halved

- 1 cucumber, sliced
- 1/2 red onion, thinly sliced
- 1/2 cup Kalamata olives, pitted
- 1/2 cup feta cheese, crumbled
- Greek dressing (store-bought or homemade)

Instructions:

1. Preheat the grill or grill pan over medium-high heat.
2. In a bowl, rub the chicken breasts with olive oil, dried oregano, salt, and pepper.
3. Grill the chicken for 6-8 minutes per side or until fully cooked. Allow it to rest for a few minutes before slicing.
4. In a large bowl, combine the salad greens, cherry tomatoes, cucumber, red onion, Kalamata olives, and feta cheese.
5. Arrange the grilled chicken slices on top of the salad.
6. Drizzle the Greek dressing over the salad or serve it on the side.
7. Toss the salad gently to combine; ensuring each bite is a medley of flavors.
8. Divide the salad between two plates and enjoy the wholesome goodness of a Greek salad with grilled chicken.

Greece's signature flavors are brought to your table with this lunchtime favorite. The grilled chicken is enhanced by the crunchy veggies, salty olives, and zesty feta, making this a filling and healthy dish that embodies the spirit of the Mediterranean diet.

5.2 Quinoa and Roasted Vegetable Bowl

Proclaimed as a superfood, quinoa takes center stage in this filling bowl full of nutrients. This recipe, when paired with a medley of roasted veggies, is a vibrant, flavorful, and nutritious feast.

Ingredients:

- 1 cup quinoa, rinsed
- 2 cups water or vegetable broth
- 2 tablespoons olive oil
- 1 cup cherry tomatoes, halved
- 1 zucchini, sliced
- 1 red bell pepper, diced
- 1 yellow bell pepper, diced
- 1 red onion, thinly sliced
- 2 cloves garlic, minced
- 1 teaspoon dried oregano
- Salt and pepper to taste
- 1/4 cup fresh basil, chopped
- 1/4 cup crumbled feta cheese (optional)

Instructions:

1. Preheat the oven to 425°F (220°C).
2. In a saucepan, combine quinoa and water or vegetable broth. Bring to a boil, then reduce heat, cover, and simmer for 15 minutes or until the quinoa is cooked and the liquid is absorbed.
3. While the quinoa is cooking, toss the cherry tomatoes, zucchini, red and yellow bell peppers, red onion, and garlic with olive oil, dried oregano, salt, and pepper.
4. Spread the vegetables on a baking sheet and roast in the preheated oven for 20-25 minutes or until the vegetables are tender and slightly caramelized.
5. Fluff the cooked quinoa with a fork and divide it between two bowls.
6. Top the quinoa with the roasted vegetables.
7. Garnish with fresh basil and crumbled feta cheese, if desired.
8. Drizzle with a touch of olive oil and season with additional salt and pepper to taste.
9. Toss the ingredients in the bowl gently before serving.

The richness of quinoa and the savory sweetness of roasted veggies come together in this delicious dish of quinoa and roasted vegetables for a great lunch alternative. It's a vibrant, nutrient-dense dish that perfectly captures the essence of the

Mediterranean diet.

5.3 Hummus Wrap with Fresh Veggies

Lunch can be enhanced with a hummus wrap stuffed with crisp veggies, providing a blast of Mediterranean flavors. This recipe makes a light and filling dinner by combining the smoothness of hummus with the crispness of fresh vegetables.

Ingredients:

- 2 large whole wheat or spinach tortillas
- 1 cup hummus (store-bought or homemade)
- 1 cucumber, julienned
- 1 carrot, julienned
- 1 bell pepper (any color), thinly sliced
- 1 cup mixed salad greens
- 1/4 cup red onion, thinly sliced
- 1/4 cup crumbled feta cheese
- Fresh lemon juice for drizzling
- Salt and pepper to taste

Instructions:

1. Lay out the tortillas on a clean surface.
2. Spread a generous layer of hummus over each tortilla.

3. Arrange the julienned cucumber, carrot, and thinly sliced bell pepper on top of the hummus.

4. Add a handful of mixed salad greens and sprinkle red onion and crumbled feta cheese over the vegetables.

5. Drizzle with fresh lemon juice and season with salt and pepper to taste.

6. Roll up the tortillas tightly to form wraps.

7. Slice each wrap in half diagonally and secure with toothpicks if needed.

8. Serve the hummus wraps immediately, and enjoy the delightful combination of textures and flavors.

This hummus wrap combines the creamy deliciousness of hummus with the freshness of vegetables for a simple and quick lunch alternative. It's the epitome of the plant-based elements and healthful simplicity of the Mediterranean Diet.

With your companion, these lunchtime favorites will take you on a culinary adventure inspired by the vibrant tapestry of flavors found throughout the Mediterranean. It's more than simply a meal. These meals are meant to fuel your bodies and your relationship, from the Greek grilled chicken to the quinoa and roasted veggies of the sun-drenched fields and the hummus wraps reflecting the lively markets. Prepare to delight in the harmony and special moments that are created with every meal, turning lunch into a celebration of spending time together and the love of cooking together.

Chapter 6: Dinner for Two

Dinner is the finish line; it's a chance to relax, tell stories, and enjoy a well-prepared meal. We explore dinners for two that capture the spirit of the Mediterranean Diet in this chapter. These dishes are not only simple and quick to prepare, but they are also intended to turn your nights into harmonious times that you can enjoy together as you travel.

6.1 Lemon Herb Salmon with Roasted Vegetables

This Lemon Herb Salmon with Roasted Vegetables highlights the flavor and health benefits of salmon, which is high in omega-3 fatty acids. This recipe, when paired with a medley of roasted veggies, is a celebration of healthful deliciousness and simplicity.

Ingredients:

- 2 salmon fillets
- 1 lemon, thinly sliced
- 2 tablespoons olive oil
- 1 tablespoon fresh dill, chopped
- 1 tablespoon fresh parsley, chopped
- Salt and pepper to taste

- 2 cups mixed vegetables (e.g., cherry tomatoes, zucchini, bell peppers, asparagus)

Instructions:

1. Preheat the oven to 400°F (200°C).
2. Place the salmon fillets on a baking sheet lined with parchment paper.
3. Drizzle olive oil over the salmon and season with salt and pepper.
4. Sprinkle chopped dill and parsley over the salmon fillets.
5. Arrange lemon slices on top of each fillet.
6. In a bowl, toss the mixed vegetables with olive oil, salt, and pepper.
7. Spread the vegetables around the salmon on the baking sheet.
8. Roast in the preheated oven for 15-20 minutes or until the salmon is cooked through and the vegetables are tender.
9. Serve the Lemon Herb Salmon over a bed of roasted vegetables and garnish with additional fresh herbs.

This romantic supper for two offers a lovely blast of zesty freshness along with a satisfying combination of heart-healthy salmon and a vibrant assortment of roasted vegetables, which is an ideal representation of the Mediterranean Diet's focus on nutrient-dense, fresh foods.

6.2 Mediterranean Stuffed Bell Peppers

A traditional and adaptable dish that is ideal for the Mediterranean diet is stuffed bell peppers. A pleasant and filling supper choice for two, these Mediterranean Stuffed Bell Peppers are packed with a savory mixture of quinoa, tomatoes, olives, and feta cheese.

Ingredients:

- 2 large bell peppers (any color)
- 1 cup cooked quinoa
- 1 cup cherry tomatoes, diced
- 1/2 cup Kalamata olives, pitted and chopped
- 1/4 cup red onion, finely chopped
- 1/4 cup feta cheese, crumbled
- 2 tablespoons fresh parsley, chopped
- 1 tablespoon olive oil
- 1 teaspoon dried oregano
- Salt and pepper to taste
- Lemon wedges for serving

Instructions:

1. Preheat the oven to 375°F (190°C).

2. Cut the bell peppers in half lengthwise, removing the seeds and membranes.

3. In a bowl, combine the cooked quinoa, cherry tomatoes, Kalamata olives, red onion, feta cheese, fresh parsley, olive oil, dried oregano, salt, and pepper.

4. Stuff each bell pepper half with the quinoa mixture, pressing it down gently.

5. Place the stuffed peppers on a baking dish and cover with aluminum foil.

6. Bake in the preheated oven for 25-30 minutes or until the peppers are tender.

7. Remove the foil and bake for an additional 5-10 minutes to allow the tops to lightly brown.

8. Serve the Mediterranean Stuffed Bell Peppers with a drizzle of olive oil and lemon wedges on the side.

Not only are these stuffed bell peppers visually stunning, but they also perfectly balance a variety of Mediterranean tastes. Quinoa, olives, tomatoes, and feta cheese combine to provide a filling, nutrient-dense supper for two.

6.3 Shrimp and Feta Pasta

This Shrimp and Feta Pasta offers a Mediterranean touch to pasta, a comfort food that's appreciated by many. This dish, which has tender shrimp, feta cheese, and a vibrant burst of cherry tomatoes, is an ode to simplicity and decadence.

Ingredients:

- 8 oz (225g) whole wheat or multigrain pasta
- 1 tablespoon olive oil
- 2 cloves garlic, minced
- 1 pound (450g) shrimp, peeled and deveined
- 1 cup cherry tomatoes, halved
- 1/2 cup crumbled feta cheese
- 2 tablespoons fresh parsley, chopped
- 1 tablespoon lemon juice
- Salt and pepper to taste
- Red pepper flakes (optional, for heat)

Instructions:

1. Cook the pasta according to package instructions until al dente. Drain and set aside.
2. In a large skillet, heat olive oil over medium heat. Add minced garlic and sauté until fragrant.
3. Add the shrimp to the skillet and cook for 2-3 minutes on each side or until they turn pink and opaque.
4. Toss in the cherry tomatoes and cook for an additional 2 minutes until they start to soften.

5. Add the cooked pasta to the skillet and toss to combine.

6. Sprinkle crumbled feta cheese over the pasta and shrimp mixture.

7. Drizzle with lemon juice and toss until the feta begins to melt and coat the pasta.

8. Season with salt, pepper, and red pepper flakes (if using).

9. Garnish with fresh parsley and serve the Shrimp and Feta Pasta hot.

The freshness of cherry tomatoes, tart feta, and succulent shrimp make for a delicious dinner for two. The dish's nutritional profile is enhanced and given a nutty flavor by the whole wheat pasta, which exemplifies the Mediterranean Diet's emphasis on balance and variety.

By creating a shared moment that goes beyond the plate, you and your companion are building an experience while you enjoy these supper recipes. Each recipe, from the colorful medley of Lemon Herb Salmon to the hearty embrace of Mediterranean Stuffed Bell Peppers and the comfortable indulgence of Shrimp and Feta Pasta, is designed to strengthen your bond and turn suppertime into a celebration of family time. With these tasty and filling dinners for two, be ready to savor the tastes of the Mediterranean as you set out on a voyage of harmony and shared moments.

Chapter 7: Shareable Side Dishes

The hidden heroes of a well-rounded dinner are the side dishes, which offer richness, complexity, and a hint of decadence. This chapter features sharing-friendly side dishes that are all influenced by the Mediterranean Diet's abundance and simplicity. These recipes are meant for two, and they will not only go well with your main courses but also improve the quality of your moments spent together as you go toward peace.

7.1 Garlic and Herb Couscous

With the addition of garlic and herbs, couscous, a mainstay of Mediterranean cuisine, becomes a tasty and aromatic side dish. This Garlic and Herb Couscous is incredibly easy to make and goes well with a wide range of main dishes.

Ingredients:

- 1 cup couscous
- 1 cup vegetable broth or water
- 2 tablespoons olive oil
- 3 cloves garlic, minced

- 1 teaspoon dried thyme

- 1 teaspoon dried rosemary

- Salt and pepper to taste

- Fresh parsley for garnish

Instructions:

1. In a saucepan, bring the vegetable broth or water to a boil.

2. Stir in the couscous, cover the saucepan, and remove it from heat. Let it sit for 5 minutes to allow the couscous to absorb the liquid.

3. Fluff the couscous with a fork to separate the grains.

4. In a separate pan, heat olive oil over medium heat.

5. Add minced garlic and sauté until fragrant, about 1-2 minutes.

6. Stir in the dried thyme and rosemary, cooking for an additional 1-2 minutes.

7. Combine the garlic and herb mixture with the fluffed couscous, tossing to distribute the flavors evenly.

8. Season with salt and pepper to taste.

9. Garnish with fresh parsley before serving.

Not only is this Garlic and Herb Couscous a delicious side dish, but it also adds a flavorful and savory touch to your family meals. Because of its simplicity, it may be served with a wide range of main courses and yet look harmonious on your dinner table.

7.2 Roasted Mediterranean Vegetables

Vegetables become more flavorful and naturally sweet when they are roasted, producing a colorful and nutrient-dense side dish. These Roasted Mediterranean Vegetables are visual and gustatory feasts that highlight the region's colorful produce.

Ingredients:

- 2 cups cherry tomatoes, halved
- 1 zucchini, sliced
- 1 yellow squash, sliced
- 1 red bell pepper, diced
- 1 yellow bell pepper, diced
- 1 red onion, thinly sliced
- 3 tablespoons olive oil
- 2 teaspoons dried oregano
- 1 teaspoon garlic powder
- Salt and pepper to taste
- Fresh basil for garnish

Instructions:

1. Preheat the oven to 425°F (220°C).

2. In a large bowl, combine the cherry tomatoes, zucchini, yellow squash, red bell pepper, yellow bell pepper, and red onion.

3. Drizzle olive oil over the vegetables and toss to coat evenly.

4. Sprinkle dried oregano, garlic powder, salt, and pepper over the vegetables, tossing again to ensure even seasoning.

5. Spread the vegetables on a baking sheet in a single layer.

6. Roast in the preheated oven for 25-30 minutes or until the vegetables are tender and caramelized, stirring halfway through.

7. Garnish with fresh basil before serving.

These Roasted Mediterranean Vegetables offer a combination of flavors that go well with a range of main meals, in addition to adding a pop of color to your plate. This side dish combines flavors that are pleasant to the eye and the mouth with luscious tomatoes, soft zucchini, and caramelized onions.

7.3 Tzatziki Sauce for Dipping

A meal with a Mediterranean flair isn't complete without tart and refreshing Tzatziki Sauce. Enjoy this adaptable dip with pita bread, grilled meats, or veggie sticks for a fantastic sharing option. Cucumber and dill give vibrant aromas and a creamy texture that make it a great addition to your recipe book.

Ingredients:

- 1 cup Greek yogurt
- 1/2 cucumber, grated and drained
- 2 cloves garlic, minced
- 1 tablespoon fresh dill, chopped
- 1 tablespoon olive oil
- 1 teaspoon lemon juice
- Salt and pepper to taste

Instructions:

1. In a bowl, combine the Greek yogurt, grated and drained cucumber, minced garlic, chopped fresh dill, olive oil, and lemon juice.
2. Mix the ingredients thoroughly until well combined.
3. Season the Tzatziki sauce with salt and pepper to taste.
4. Refrigerate the sauce for at least 30 minutes to allow the flavors to meld.
5. Before serving, garnish with additional chopped dill and a drizzle of olive oil if desired.

Tzatziki Sauce gives your meals a zesty, refreshing touch. It goes well with grilled meats and veggies, or it can be served as a cool dip for a variety of appetizers. Its rich flavors and creamy texture enhance your eating experience while bringing a hint of Mediterranean flair to your special occasions.

By include these side dishes in your family's dinners, you're not only bringing out the tastes on your table but also fostering a Mediterranean Diet-inspired dining atmosphere. Not only are the Roasted Mediterranean Vegetables, Garlic and Herb Couscous, and Tzatziki Sauce for Dipping accompaniments, but they are vital components that enhance the harmony and shared delight of your culinary adventure. Prepare to savor the ease and sophistication of these side dishes as you carry on your journey of companionship and the delight of cooking together.

Chapter 8: Sweet Endings

A shared meal would not be complete without a sweet ending, a chance to savor the delights of dessert. This chapter has delicious finales meant for two, many of which are influenced by the delectable and wholesome treats of the Mediterranean diet. These delicious treats are designed to bring a hint of sweetness to your moments spent together while you work toward harmony. They are also quick and simple to prepare.

8.1 Berry and Yogurt Parfait

A tasty way to embrace the freshness and vibrancy of Mediterranean cuisine and end your meal on a sweet note is with a Berry and Yogurt Parfait. The sweetness of berries and the smoothness of yogurt combine in this straightforward yet elegant dessert to create a parfait that is both aesthetically pleasing and delectable.

Ingredients:

- 1 cup mixed berries (strawberries, blueberries, raspberries)
- 1 cup Greek yogurt

- 2 tablespoons honey
- 1/2 cup granola
- Mint leaves for garnish (optional)

Instructions:

1. In serving glasses or bowls, start with a layer of Greek yogurt.
2. Add a layer of mixed berries on top of the yogurt.
3. Drizzle honey over the berries for a touch of sweetness.
4. Sprinkle a layer of granola over the berries.
5. Repeat the layers until you reach the top of the glass.
6. Garnish with a few fresh berries and mint leaves, if desired.

Serve the Berry and Yogurt Parfait immediately, savoring the layers of textures and flavors.

In addition to satisfying your sweet tooth, this Berry and Yogurt Parfait delivers a healthy dose of antioxidants from the colorful berries and the beneficial probiotics in the Greek yogurt. It's a cool, light dessert that gives your special moments a splash of color.

8.2 Olive Oil and Orange Cake

An essential ingredient in Mediterranean cooking, olive oil becomes a rich and savory cake when combined with the zesty brightness of oranges. This cake with olive oil and orange juice is a celebration of basic components that come together to make a healthy yet decadent dessert.

Ingredients:

- 1 cup all-purpose flour
- 1/2 cup almond flour
- 1 teaspoon baking powder
- 1/2 teaspoon baking soda
- 1/4 teaspoon salt
- 1/2 cup olive oil
- 1/2 cup honey
- 2 large eggs
- 1 teaspoon vanilla extract
- Zest of 1 orange
- 1/2 cup fresh orange juice
- Powdered sugar for dusting (optional)

Instructions:

1. Preheat the oven to 350°F (180°C). Grease and flour a cake pan.
2. In a bowl, whisk together the all-purpose flour, almond flour, baking powder, baking soda, and salt.
3. In a separate bowl, whisk together the olive oil, honey, eggs, vanilla extract, orange zest, and fresh orange juice until well combined.
4. Gradually add the dry ingredients to the wet ingredients, mixing until just combined.
5. Pour the batter into the prepared cake pan.
6. Bake in the preheated oven for 25-30 minutes or until a toothpick inserted into the center comes out clean.
7. Allow the cake to cool in the pan for 10 minutes before transferring it to a wire rack to cool completely.
8. Dust the Olive Oil and Orange Cake with powdered sugar before serving, if desired.

The delightful balance of sweetness and zesty freshness is achieved in this Olive Oil and Orange Cake. Olive oil gives the cake a distinct depth of flavor and makes it moist and tender. It's the ideal way to finish your dinner with a slice of decadent Mediterranean cake.

8.3 Dark Chocolate-Dipped Strawberries

Strawberries and dark chocolate are a classic pairing that combines the natural sweetness of ripe berries with the richness of chocolate. These Dark Chocolate-Dipped Strawberries are a simple yet sophisticated way to bring a little decadence into your moments together.

Ingredients:

- 1 cup dark chocolate chips
- 1 tablespoon coconut oil
- 1 pint fresh strawberries, washed and dried

Instructions:

1. In a heatproof bowl, melt the dark chocolate chips and coconut oil together, either in a microwave or using a double boiler.
2. Stir the chocolate mixture until smooth and well combined.
3. Hold each strawberry by the stem and dip it into the melted chocolate, ensuring it's coated halfway.
4. Place the dipped strawberries on a parchment-lined tray.
5. Allow the chocolate to set by placing the tray in the refrigerator for 15-20 minutes.

6. Once the chocolate is firm, serve the Dark Chocolate-Dipped Strawberries on a platter.

These indulgent treats not only satisfy your sweet tooth but also provide a dose of antioxidants from the dark chocolate and the nutritional benefits of fresh strawberries. The combination of the velvety chocolate coating and the juicy sweetness of the strawberries create a harmonious and irresistible dessert.

As you share these sweet endings with your partner, you're not just enjoying a dessert; you're creating a memorable conclusion to your shared meals. The Berry and Yogurt Parfait, Olive Oil and Orange Cake, and Dark Chocolate-Dipped Strawberries are more than just recipes they're a testament to the simplicity and richness of Mediterranean desserts. Get ready to savor the sweetness of these moments and celebrate the joy of cooking as a couple on your journey to harmony.

Chapter 9: Snack Time Treats

Snack time is an opportunity to rejuvenate and share a moment of enjoyment with your partner. In this chapter, we explore delightful and healthy snacks designed for two, inspired by the Mediterranean Diet. These recipes are not only quick and easy but also crafted to add a burst of flavor to your shared moments on the journey to harmony.

9.1 Mediterranean Trail Mix

Trail mix is a versatile and energizing snack that perfectly aligns with the principles of the Mediterranean Diet. This Mediterranean Trail Mix combines a mix of nuts, seeds, and dried fruits, creating a snack that is not only satisfying but also rich in nutrients.

Ingredients:

- 1 cup almonds
- 1 cup walnuts
- 1/2 cup pumpkin seeds
- 1/2 cup dried apricots, chopped
- 1/2 cup dried cranberries
- 1 teaspoon olive oil

- 1 teaspoon honey

- 1 teaspoon dried oregano

- 1/2 teaspoon sea salt

Instructions:

1. Preheat the oven to 350°F (180°C).

2. In a bowl, toss the almonds, walnuts, and pumpkin seeds with olive oil, honey, dried oregano, and sea salt until evenly coated.

3. Spread the nut and seed mixture on a baking sheet in a single layer.

4. Roast in the preheated oven for 10-12 minutes or until the nuts are golden brown, stirring halfway through.

5. Allow the trail mix to cool completely before adding the dried apricots and cranberries.

6. Toss everything together and transfer the Mediterranean Trail Mix to an airtight container.

This trail mix not only provides a satisfying crunch but also incorporates the flavors of the Mediterranean with the addition of oregano. It's a snack that's as nutritious as it is delicious, perfect for refueling and sharing a moment of togetherness.

9.2 Roasted Red Pepper Hummus with Pita

Hummus, a classic Mediterranean dip, takes on a flavorful twist with the addition of roasted red peppers. This Roasted Red Pepper Hummus with Pita is a savory and satisfying snack that is both easy to prepare and perfect for sharing.

Ingredients:

- 1 can (15 oz) chickpeas, drained and rinsed
- 1/2 cup roasted red peppers, drained
- 1/4 cup tahini
- 2 cloves garlic
- 2 tablespoons olive oil
- 1 tablespoon lemon juice
- 1/2 teaspoon ground cumin
- Salt and pepper to taste
- Fresh parsley for garnish
- Pita bread for serving

Instructions:

1. In a food processor, combine the chickpeas, roasted red peppers, tahini, garlic, olive oil, lemon juice, ground cumin, salt, and pepper.

2. Blend the ingredients until smooth, scraping down the sides as needed.

3. If the hummus is too thick, add a little water, one tablespoon at a time, until you reach your desired consistency.

4. Transfer the hummus to a serving bowl and drizzle with olive oil.

5. Garnish with fresh parsley.

6. Serve the Roasted Red Pepper Hummus with Pita bread for dipping.

This hummus variation adds a burst of color and a hint of smokiness to the classic chickpea dip. Paired with warm pita bread, it's a snack that encourages sharing, making it a delightful addition to your moments of relaxation.

9.3 Feta and Olive Stuffed Cherry Tomatoes

Cherry tomatoes, with their juicy sweetness, serve as the perfect vessel for a savory and flavorful stuffing. These Feta and Olive Stuffed Cherry Tomatoes are a quick and easy snack that combines the brininess of olives with the creamy richness of feta cheese.

Ingredients:

- 1 pint cherry tomatoes
- 1/2 cup feta cheese, crumbled
- 1/4 cup Kalamata olives, pitted and chopped
- 2 tablespoons fresh basil, chopped
- 1 tablespoon olive oil
- Salt and pepper to taste

Instructions:

1. Cut a small slice off the top of each cherry tomato to create a flat base.
2. Use a small spoon or melon baller to scoop out the seeds and create a hollow space in each tomato.
3. In a bowl, combine the crumbled feta cheese, chopped Kalamata olives, fresh basil, and olive oil. Mix well.
4. Season the filling with salt and pepper to taste.
5. Stuff each cherry tomato with the feta and olive mixture, pressing it gently to pack the stuffing.
6. Arrange the stuffed cherry tomatoes on a serving platter.
7. Drizzle with a little extra olive oil and garnish with additional fresh basil.
8. Serve these Feta and Olive Stuffed Cherry Tomatoes as a refreshing and savory snack.

These bite-sized treats not only showcase the vibrant colors of the

Mediterranean but also bring together the bold flavors of feta and olives. The combination of juicy tomatoes and savory stuffing creates a snack that's both satisfying and perfect for sharing during moments of relaxation.

As you indulge in these snack time treats with your partner, you're not just enjoying a quick bite; you're savoring the flavors of the Mediterranean and enhancing your shared moments. The Mediterranean Trail Mix, Roasted Red Pepper Hummus with Pita, and Feta and Olive Stuffed Cherry Tomatoes are not just snacks they're a celebration of simplicity, health, and the joy of snacking together. Get ready to enjoy these delightful treats as you continue your journey to harmony and the joy of cooking as a couple.

Chapter 10: Drinks for Two

Without a cool drink to go with it, a well-balanced lunch is incomplete. This chapter features simple and delicious beverages that are perfect for a couple and are influenced by the Mediterranean diet. In addition to being easy to make, these recipes are designed to infuse your shared moments on the path to harmony with flavor and moisture.

10.1 Citrus-Infused Water

Drinking plenty of water is important, and there's no better way to stay hydrated than with tasty and pleasant citrus-infused water. Not only does this refreshing drink soothe your thirst, but it also gives your shared meals a hint of Mediterranean brightness.

Ingredients:

- 1 orange, thinly sliced
- 1 lemon, thinly sliced
- 1 lime, thinly sliced
- 1 handful fresh mint leaves
- Ice cubes
- 4 cups water

Instructions:

1. In a pitcher, combine the sliced orange, lemon, and lime.
2. Add fresh mint leaves to the pitcher.
3. Fill the pitcher with ice cubes.
4. Pour 4 cups of water over the ice and citrus slices.
5. Stir gently to combine the ingredients.
6. Let the Citrus-Infused Water sit in the refrigerator for at least 30 minutes to allow the flavors to meld.
7. Serve the refreshing drink in glasses, garnishing with additional mint leaves if desired.

This citrus-infused water not only keeps you hydrated but also infuses your conversations with a zesty, invigorating burst of citrus flavor. Oranges, lemons, limes, and mint come together to make a refreshing drink that goes well with any meal and is a great addition to your repertoire of beverages for two.

10.2 Herbal Iced Tea with Mint

A traditional and adaptable beverage, iced tea takes on a fragrant and energizing quality when it is flavored with herbs like mint. This Mint Herbal Iced Tea is the ideal complement to your social gatherings, providing a tasty and calming way to improve your mealtime experience.

Ingredients:

- 2 herbal tea bags (such as chamomile, peppermint, or your favorite herbal blend)
- 4 cups boiling water
- 1 tablespoon honey (optional)
- Fresh mint leaves for garnish
- Ice cubes

Instructions:

1. Place the herbal tea bags in a heatproof pitcher.
2. Pour boiling water over the tea bags.
3. Allow the tea too steep for 5-7 minutes, or as directed on the tea bag.
4. Remove the tea bags and discard them.
5. Stir in honey, if desired, while the tea is still warm.
6. Let the tea cool to room temperature, then refrigerate for at least 1 hour.
7. Serve the Herbal Iced Tea over ice, garnished with fresh mint leaves.

In addition to being a delicious take on a classic iced tea, this Herbal Iced Tea with Mint offers the relaxing and aromatic properties of herbal infusions. It's a tasty and nutritious garnish for your cocktails for two, bringing a little peace to your moments together.

10.3 Pomegranate and Basil Sparkler

A Pomegranate and Basil Sparkler, which combines the herbal freshness of basil with the sweet-tart tones of pomegranate, will elevate your drinking experience. This vibrant, eye-catching beverage is a feast for the senses and goes great with your shared meals.

Ingredients:

- 1 cup pomegranate juice
- 2 tablespoons fresh basil leaves, chopped
- 1 tablespoon honey
- Sparkling water
- Ice cubes
- Pomegranate seeds and basil leaves for garnish

Instructions:

1. In a glass, combine pomegranate juice, chopped basil, and honey.
2. Stir well to dissolve the honey and infuse the flavors.

3. Fill the glass with ice cubes.

4. Top the mixture with sparkling water, leaving some space at the top for fizz.

5. Stir gently to combine the ingredients.

6. Garnish with pomegranate seeds and a sprig of basil.

7. Serve the Pomegranate and Basil Sparkler immediately, enjoying the effervescence and burst of flavors.

This bubbly not only elevates your special moments together but also combines the distinct flavors of basil and pomegranate. The fizz of sparkling water adds a wonderful touch to your drinks for two, elevating the whole experience.

Enjoying these drinks for two will do more for you than just keep you hydrated the bright aromas of the Mediterranean will elevate your moments spent together. More than just drinks, the Citrus-Infused Water, Pomegranate and Basil Sparkler, and Herbal Iced Tea with Mint are celebrations of simplicity, freshness, and the delight of sharing a drink with others. Prepare to toast to the harmony and moments spent together that these beverages will offer to your gastronomic adventure. Drinks!

Chapter 11: Tips for Cooking and Eating Together

Taking a culinary adventure together can be a fulfilling experience that extends beyond cooking together. We'll go over some basic cooking and dining tips in this chapter, with a focus on teamwork, communication, and the happiness that comes from making mealtimes a treasured and peaceful part of your bond.

11.1 Communication in the Kitchen

Effective communication is essential for any successful team effort, and this also holds true in the kitchen. Meal preparation can become a smooth and joyful experience if you and your partner can communicate well while cooking.

1. Talk about Preferences and Dietary Needs: Before going to the kitchen, discuss each other's dietary requirements and preferences. Knowing the tastes and ingredients that you both appreciate will help you select recipes that suit your palates.

2. Plan Meals Together: Spend some time working together to organize your meals. Together, create a grocery list by talking about the meals you want to attempt and taking into account the supplies you already have. In the kitchen, preparation ahead of time can save time and ease tension.

3. Assign Roles and Tasks: To expedite the cooking process, clearly identify roles and tasks. Separating tasks between two people guarantees efficiency and keeps the kitchen from becoming chaotic, whether one person concentrates on slicing vegetables while the other handles the stove.

4. Keep Lines of Communication Open: When cooking, keep lines of communication open. Take suggestions, give ideas, and enjoy the process with one another. Good communication makes both of you feel like you're part of the culinary creation and encourages teamwork.

5. Remember to Thank Each Other: It's important to let each other know how much you appreciate their efforts. In the kitchen, a simple "thank you" can go a long way toward fostering a friendly and upbeat environment.

11.2 Dividing and Conquering Tasks

Cooking together involves sharing tasks to enhance efficiency and enjoyment in addition to food preparation. The following advice can help you divide and conquer kitchen tasks:

1. Determine Preferences and Strengths: Acknowledge each other's advantages and preferences in the kitchen. Let the person who enjoys grilling handle the barbecue while the other person concentrates on making salads or other side dishes. Assigning responsibilities according to preferences guarantees that both partners are involved and content in their jobs.

2. Make a Cooking Schedule: Make a cooking schedule that alternates who is in charge of the kitchen. This guarantees an equitable allocation of responsibilities and affords every individual a chance to demonstrate their culinary prowess.

3. Work in Parallel: Try to complete several meal components at the same time. One person can cook the main course and the other can take care of the dessert and side dishes. Simultaneous operation expedites the cooking process and reduces idle time.

4. Alternate duties Occasionally: You might spice up your culinary routine by alternating duties. If one individual usually takes the lead, consider rotating positions from time to time. This allows both spouses to enjoy the various facets of cooking while also keeping things interesting.

5. Assign Clean up Tasks: Cleaning up after a meal is a crucial step in the cooking process. Whether it's putting materials away, cleaning countertops, or washing dishes, divide up the clean-up duties. Cooking is a collaborative activity, which is reinforced when clean-up is done jointly.

11.3 Making Cooking a Bonding Experience

It takes more than just preparing food to turn cooking into a bonding activity; it's about making enduring memories and spending time together. Here's how to turn cooking into a fun activity that you do together:

1. Together, choose recipes: This can be an enjoyable and cooperative exercise. Look through recipe books, web resources, or even compile a list of common recipes. By selecting recipes together, you can make sure that both spouses are enthusiastic about the meals you'll be cooking.

2. Establish a Calm Atmosphere: Lighten the mood in the kitchen by establishing a calm environment. Pour a glass of wine, light some lights, or play your favorite music. A good cooking experience is enhanced by a cozy and entertaining setting.

3. Play and Experiment: Don't be scared to play around with flavors and substances. Playing about in the kitchen is a great opportunity when cooking together. Together, experiment with different methods and ingredients, and relish the process of creating delicious new dishes.

4. Tell Tales and Have Meaningful Conversations: Make the most of your cooking time by telling stories and having deep discussions. In the kitchen, people may connect and communicate about everything from future plans to favorite dishes in the past.

5. Honor accomplishments: Honor your culinary accomplishments, no matter how modest. Respect one another's efforts, whether it's trying a new recipe and succeeding or mastering a difficult dish. In the kitchen, joy and a sense of success are fostered by positive reinforcement.

As soon as the food is ready, set a table that is shared by all. Make the eating experience an extension of your cooking efforts by paying attention to presentation and attentively arranging the food. It becomes the result of your combined efforts when you sit down to eat together.

Together, cooking and dining can be a joyful, educational, and intimate experience. Along with making delicious meals, you and your partner are strengthening your bond by emphasizing effective communication, thoughtfully allocating tasks, and making cooking a fun activity. Savor the moments of companionship and the peaceful experience of sharing a meal made with love and teamwork as you continue on this culinary adventure.

Chapter 12: Conclusion

12.1 Celebrating Your Culinary Journey

When you finish this cookbook, stop to consider the culinary adventures you and your partner have shared. Savor the tastes, the times spent together, and the happiness that cooking has brought into your lives. Every recipe you've looked at was created with the simplicity and richness of the Mediterranean Diet in mind, providing a feast for the senses in addition to providing body nourishment.

You've learned the power of five basic ingredients that are thoughtfully chosen to bring out the best flavors of Mediterranean cuisine while preparing these quick and delicious dishes. Every recipe was created to elevate your culinary experience and create memorable moments with friends and family, whether it was the zesty Citrus-Infused Water, the fragrant Herbal Iced Tea with Mint, or the savory Feta and Olive Stuffed Cherry Tomatoes.

12.2 The Path to Harmony and Shared Moments

Cooking and dining together is a journey toward harmony and

special times spent together, not just a ritual. The idea behind this cookbook is that cooking together and sharing meals is a great way to deepen your relationship. With its focus on healthful, fresh foods, the Mediterranean diet not only nourishes your bodies but also promotes tastings of different flavors and textures with others.

You've embraced careful work division, good communication in the kitchen, and turning cooking into a fun way to bond with others. All of these actions have put you on the path to harmony. Not only are the recipes a compilation of foods, but they also serve as a tribute to the joy, richness, and simplicity inherent in the practice of cooking together.

Continue to celebrate your gastronomic adventure as you go. Taste new foods, experiment with flavors, and cherish the times you spend with your family in the kitchen. Keep in mind that eating together is a celebration of your relationship, a chance to bond, and a chance to make enduring memories. It's not just about eating.

I hope the times you spend together at the table are full of joy, merriment, and the satisfaction of cooking a great dinner. Not merely a cookbook, The Easy 5-Ingredient Mediterranean Diet Cookbook for Two is an encouragement to carry on exploring the food world together, promoting harmony, and savoring the pleasure of cooking together.

I appreciate you joining me on this delicious journey. Cheers too many more dinners together, fun new adventures, and the timeless pleasure of cooking together. Cheers to good food and cooking!

About the Author

Dr. Adam C. stands as a beacon of inspiration in the fields of medicine, nutrition, and self-help, with a remarkable journey that exemplifies the transformative power of healthy living. Armed with a professional master's degree in health nutrition and years of experience, Dr. C. has become a guiding light for individuals seeking to embrace vibrant well-being and lead happier lives.

From an early age, Dr. C. navigated through a myriad of health challenges that ranged from genetic predispositions to the pitfalls of unhealthy eating. His personal struggle ignited a flame of determination within him, one that was fueled by the belief that the human body possesses an incredible ability to heal and rejuvenate through the right nourishment. Through steadfast dedication, Dr. C. managed to conquer his own ailments and emerged as a living testament to the transformative potential of a well-balanced lifestyle.

What sets Dr. Adam C. apart is his rich tapestry of experiences, having been deeply immersed in groundbreaking research in health food and diet-related domains. His quest to uncover the hidden treasures of nutrients within our meals has led to groundbreaking revel actions that empower individuals to extract the maximum benefit from their dietary choices. Dr. C.'s research has not only contributed to the scientific community but has also served as a roadmap for countless individuals striving to optimize their health.

However, it is not just Dr. C.'s academic prowess that has touched lives it is his unparalleled compassion and empathy that truly make him a beacon of hope. His personal journey of triumph over adversity infuses his guidance with an authentic understanding of the challenges his readers and patients face. Dr. C. doesn't just prescribe nutritional plans; he fosters a deep connection with his audience, instilling in them the confidence to embark on their own transformative journeys.

Dr. Adam C.'s holistic approach reaches beyond the confines of traditional medicine. His insights have translated into self-help resources that empower individuals to take charge of their wellness narrative. His words resonate on paper as they do in person, making his books not mere guides, but trusted companions on the path to vitality.

In the realm of health and nutrition, Dr. C. shines as a true luminary. His core strengths lie in his ability to synthesize complex scientific findings into practical, actionable advice that individuals from all walks of life can seamlessly integrate into their routines. Dr. C.'s legacy is not just a collection of breakthroughs; it is a testament to the extraordinary potential that lies within each of us to overcome obstacles and embrace a life brimming with health, happiness, and fulfillment.

As an experienced doctor, passionate nutritionist, and empathetic author, Dr. Adam C. continues to transform lives, showing us that the journey to a healthier, happier existence is within our grasp, waiting to be unlocked through the power of informed choices and unwavering determination.

www.ingramcontent.com/pod-product-compliance
Lightning Source LLC
Chambersburg PA
CBHW050842260726
48660CB00006B/2393